Dianelis Montes de Oca Cruz
Jeraldine Jiménez Cabrera
Damaris Katina López Hérnandez

Retention of permanent anterior teeth

Dianelis Montes de Oca Cruz
Jeraldine Jiménez Cabrera
Damaris Katina López Hérnandez

Retention of permanent anterior teeth

Behavior in children and adolescents

ScienciaScripts

Imprint

Cover image: www.ingimage.com

This book is a translation from the original published under ISBN 978-613-9-44149-5.

Publisher:
Sciencia Scripts
is a trademark of
Dodo Books Indian Ocean Ltd. and OmniScriptum S.R.L publishing group

120 High Road, East Finchley, London, N2 9ED, United Kingdom
Str. Armeneasca 28/1, office 1, Chisinau MD-2012, Republic of Moldova, Europe
Printed at: see last page
ISBN: 978-620-8-26015-6

Title:

Retention of permanent anterior teeth
Behaviour in the paediatric and juvenile population

Authors:

Dr. Dianelis Montes de Oca Cruz. Basic General Stomatologist.

Second year resident in General Comprehensive Stomatology.

Dr. Yeraldine Jiménez Cabrera.

First degree specialist in General Comprehensive Stomatology.
First degree specialist
in Orthodontics. Assistant Professor. MSc. in Odontostomatology for children and adolescents.

Damarys Katina López Hernández
Degree in Stomatological Care. Assistant Professor at UCM

2024

SUMMARY

Introduction: Retained teeth are those that, when the normal eruption period arrives, remain enclosed within the maxilla or mandible, maintaining the integrity of their physiological pericoronary sac. General objective: To characterise the retention of permanent anterior teeth in students between 8 and 19 years of age from schools who attended orthodontic consultations at the Manuel Fajardo Polyclinic in Santo Domingo. Methodology: A descriptive, cross-sectional study was carried out in the orthodontic clinic of the Santo Domingo polyclinic from January 2023 to March 2024. The population consisted of all students aged 8 to 19 years from the schools who attended the clinic and were diagnosed with retained permanent anterior teeth, 67 cases of which were counted. Variables: Age, sex, retained tooth, location, position, cause and treatment. Results: The most affected sex was male. The mean age of the females was 12.1 years and of the males 11.4 years. The canines were the teeth most frequently found to be impacted. The vestibular position was the most frequent. Persistence of the temporomandibular was the main cause. The majority treatment was tooth extraction. Conclusions: In the population studied, retention of permanent anterior teeth predominated in males. Canines were the most affected in the vestibular position. Temporal impaction was the most common cause and the most frequent treatment was tooth extraction.

Keywords: causes, permanent anterior teeth, position, retention, treatment.

INDEX

INTRODUCTION

The World Health Organisation (WHO) defines retained teeth as those that, once the normal eruption period has arrived, remain enclosed within the maxilla or mandible, maintaining the integrity of their physiological perichorionic sac. [1]

The incidence of tooth retention ranges from 8-14% of the general population. Any permanent, temporary or supernumerary tooth can be retained, although it occurs less frequently in the case of temporary teeth than in permanent teeth. The most affected teeth include upper and lower third molars, upper canines, lower second premolars and supernumerary teeth. However, the most important from an aesthetic and functional point of view are the upper canines and upper central incisors.[2]

There are multiple causes involved in dental retention, including local causes such as: the density of the bone covering the tooth, lack of space in the micrognathic maxilla and mandible, prolonged retention or premature loss of primary teeth, gingival fibrosis, etc. General or systemic causes include: malnutrition, rickets, anaemia, endocrine-metabolic disorders, among others. Canines, being the last teeth to appear in the group of teeth in the maxillary anterior area, also have a high incidence of becoming trapped or developing an ectopic eruption, which compromises the patient's overall health and aesthetics.[3]

Early diagnosis by means of diagnostic aids (X-rays, CT scans) is essential, as dental impaction can cause lesions such as root resorption of adjacent roots, tooth displacement, pericoronaritis, abscesses, among others. Management and treatment options depend on the type of impaction, its severity and the age of the patient.[4]

A prevalence of impacted teeth of 10.8 % is reported in China, higher than in Turkey, where 6.15 % is reported, with a prevalence in the maxilla and female sex. In Latin America and the Caribbean, the figures are higher, with 15.1 % in Colombia and 45.5 % in Cuba.[5]

Díaz[6] , in an investigation carried out in 2018 at the University of Seville, Spain, entitled: "Horizontally retained central incisor. Clinical management", found that the frequency of retained central incisors in the maxilla varied between 0.06% and 2%, causing a condition that affected facial aesthetics.

Marquez and Soto[7] , in their study "Tratamiento ortodóncico en paciente con caninos retenidos", published in the journal Tamé, Mexico, reported that impacted canines can lead to cysts, infection and migration of neighbouring teeth.

In Santiago de Cuba, it has been published that between 70.7 % and 86.9 % of the inhabitants of the territory have at least one tooth of this type retained, to which must be added the great mestization existing in the area, which favours the existence of bone-tooth discrepancies due to the combination of characteristics of one racial group and another.[5]

In the research carried out in the city of Cienfuegos, the main objective of which was to characterise patients with retained teeth with a sample of 107 patients, it was found that the most affected age group was between 14 and 17 years of age and 75% of patients with retained supernumerary teeth were located in the maxilla in the midline. The remaining 25% were located in the lower bicuspid region and upper canine region. [2]

Rodríguez et al.8 carried out a study in Villa Clara in 2021, which they called "Dental retention of the upper right central incisor due to compound odontoma", which was treated by surgical excision of the tumour and bonding of the retained right central incisor by epidental means with brackets.

In Villa Clara there is other research on retained permanent anterior teeth, including a clinical case in the Arnaldo Milián Castro hospital in Santa Clara, where two supernumerary teeth were observed causing retention of the upper central incisor and upper right canine.[9]

On carrying out the Health Situation Analysis, an increase in dental alterations was identified in school-age patients, particularly the retention of permanent anterior teeth. We were motivated to investigate the characteristics of this anomaly, given that it is a phenomenon that can affect aesthetics and function in individuals and is a reason for consultation, in addition to the fact that timely diagnosis and treatment at the first level of care would avoid more costly interventions and more costly technology. Despite being so common, there was no evidence of previous research on this topic in the municipality.

Scientific problem: What were the characteristics of the retention of permanent anterior teeth in students aged 8 to 19 years who attended the orthodontic clinic of the Santo Domingo Polyclinic?

GENERAL OBJECTIVE:

To characterise the retention of permanent anterior teeth in students aged 8 to 19 years from schools attending the orthodontic clinic of the Manuel Piti Fajardo Polyclinic in Santo Domingo.

SPECIFIC OBJECTIVES:

1. To characterise the population studied according to socio-demographic variables.
2. Identify the location and position of retained permanent anterior teeth.
3. To determine the causes of tooth retention in this population.
4. To determine the treatment for tooth retention in the patients under study.
5. Relate the possible association of sex with retention position and treatment.

THEORETICAL FRAMEWORK

Tooth retention

The World Health Organisation (WHO) defines retained teeth as those that, once the normal eruption period has arrived, remain enclosed within the maxilla or mandible, maintaining the integrity of their physiological pericoronary sac. It is the failure to exfoliate at the indicated time, with the consequent alteration in the eruption of the substitute.[1, 10]

Tooth eruption starts from the embryological formation of the tooth until its eruption into the oral cavity. It is considered a dynamic and physiological event that influences the development of the stomatognathic apparatus and the growth of the craniofacial structures.[11]

It occurs in response to various factors such as root growth, alveolar bone growth, muscular action, alveolar ridge resorption, and reorganisation of the alveolar ligament. In most cases, this process helps to establish correct occlusion.[12]

Each of these aspects means that dental eruption has its own characteristics in each subject, so that the chronology of dental emergence is relatively variable. On certain occasions, there is a delay in this physiological mechanism, which is called "late eruption", which is defined as "a scarce eruption of the tooth despite having an unobstructed path for its correct position in the oral cavity".[13]

Phases of tooth eruption

The process of tooth eruption is composed of three phases, which in chronological order are:

a) Pre-eruptive phase: This stage is comprised of the rupture of the pedicle that triggers the differentiation of the tooth germ until the development of the crown is complete. This pre-eruptive displacement and adaptations on the part of the supporting structures allow the tooth germs to obtain the correct position within the jaws. Although at the beginning there is an extremely small space between germ and germ, it is the necessary stimulus for the basal bones to expand in all directions giving the exact dimensions for the balance between them. Therefore, it can be said that the movement of the germs is also resolved by the osteoclastic or remodelling activity of the bone tissue, as it occurs at the same time as the tooth is being formed.

b) Pre-functional eruptive phase: This phase comprises the eruption of the tooth after its formation. Therefore, the tooth is immersed in the basal bones in the development phase to begin its route towards the occlusal plane adapting its respective position, i.e. the migration of the tooth in the apical direction of the gingiva and gingival sulcus occurs until it occludes with its antagonist. Furthermore, this stage includes ligament formation, which occurs after root formation, and what is important to mention is that the synthesis and degradation of these fibres by fibroblasts facilitates the eruption of the teeth. Having said this, it can be stated that it is at this stage that an area of reddening of the oral mucosa is noted, which subsequently becomes ischemic and produces the union of the oral epithelium with the dental epithelium, so that an active movement of the jawbone, also called "active eruption", and at the same time an apical movement of the gingival soft tissues, also called "passive eruption", is carried out.

c) Functional eruptive phase: This includes the instant when the tooth comes into contact with its antagonist and then stops its vertical displacement, until the exfoliation of the primary dentition takes place. Even so, the movements that occur at this stage are mainly because the tooth continues to adapt throughout its life to compensate for its own wear and tear and the forces to which it is exposed.[13] , 14, [15]

Eruption sequence in the permanent dentition

The eruption of the permanent dentition begins at six years of age. In the maxilla, the sequence begins with the emergence of the first molar, followed by the central incisors, then the lateral incisors, the first premolar, second premolar and then the canines and second molar.

In the mandible, it is relatively similar, as eruption begins with the first molar, then the central incisors and then the lateral incisors, however, the difference lies in the fact that the next tooth to emerge is the canine followed by the first premolar, second premolar and second permanent lower molar. It is necessary to emphasise that "with regard to the sequence of eruption, it has been observed that, although there is a general pattern, not all individuals obey the same sequence".[16]

As a counterpart to the eruption process, there is also dental inclusion, which Gil de la Serna et al.[17] define as the eruptive pathological process whereby the tooth fails to erupt through the buccal mucosa, and consequently does not achieve a functional position in the dental arch.

It should be taken into account that inclusion, impaction and retention are not synonymous; therefore, an included tooth is one that remains in the bone and inclusion encompasses dental retentions and impactions. We can distinguish between ectopic inclusion, when the included tooth is in an anomalous position but close to its usual location, and heterotopic inclusion, when the tooth is in an anomalous position further away from its usual location. A tooth is considered to be retained when it has not taken its place in the arch beyond the age of eruption.[18], [19]

Incidence of dental impaction

women. 20,21, 22

Retention of incisors is most common in the upper jaw. Its incidence in the population is approximately 0.1-0.5%. Retention of the upper canine affects 0.8-2.9% of the population. It is more frequent in females and in 85% of cases the retention is palatal. The upper canines are one of the last teeth to erupt in the maxilla and space for them may be compromised in the dental arch at the time of eruption. On the other hand, retention of the lower canine is quite rare, ranging from 0.05 to 0.04%. Forty percent of the cases seem to be related to a malformation, malposition or agenesis of the permanent lateral. The most frequent position is palatal. The canines are considered the most important teeth of the stomatognathic system being indispensable for the functional movements of laterality and protrusion responsible for function, occlusal harmony and aesthetics. The retention of premolars is approximately 0.3% for mandibular premolars and 0.2% for maxillary premolars. For first and second molars it is approximately 0.02% for upper first molars and 0.08% for upper second molars. For lower molars, the frequency is 0.04% for lower first molars and 0.06% for lower second molars. Finally, the incidence of retention of third molars is approximately 20-30%, with a certain preponderance in the lower first molars and 0.06% in the upper second molars.

Causes of tooth retention

The aetiopathogenesis of dental eruption anomalies is not completely known. The fact of this peculiar abnormality of tooth eruption must be sought in its first cause, in the very origin of the human species. Anthropologists state that the cerebration of the human being, constantly increasing, except in significant cases, enlarges his cranial cavity at the expense of the jaws. The prehypophyseal line which sloped forward from the receding forehead to the protruding jaw in pre-human forms has become almost vertical in modern man as the number of teeth has decreased.[23]

Tooth retention increases with the evolution of the human being, given the involution that the maxilla and mandible are undergoing, which is due, among other causes, to the change in diet experienced in recent centuries and the trend towards a softer and more refined diet, which makes a more powerful masticatory apparatus unnecessary. The different parts that make up the stomatognathic apparatus have decreased in inverse proportion to their hardness and plasticity, i.e. the muscles have decreased in size the most, because the masticatory function has decreased, followed by the bones and finally the teeth. The eruption of permanent teeth obeys the same biological laws as the primary dentition. Independently of the phylogenetic predisposing causes of dental inclusion, which cannot be controlled despite our knowledge of them, there are other processes that favour this alteration. In general, this anomaly has a complex aetiology that is preceded by evolutionary, anatomical and mechanical factors.[24], [25]

Genetic or systemic factors such as endocrine disorders, febrile conditions and irradiation are involved in this pathology. It is also related to metabolism, congenital ectodermal polydysplasia and osteoporosis.[26]

Various local causes have also been identified such as: bone-tooth discrepancies; root dilacerations; early loss or prolonged retention of the deciduous canine; ankylosis; cysts; presence of supernumerary teeth; premature apex closure; trauma; and iatrogenesis. In addition to the above, there are also predetermining factors that influence the occurrence of impacted teeth, such as the patient's age, gender or systemic history. All of these co-factors are associated with the severity of tooth retention, which may influence future problems such as misalignment of adjacent teeth or occlusal failure. [27]

Causal factors can be classified as local and systemic:

Local factors:

These include the irregular position of the tooth or pressure from an adjacent tooth, which could be due to the anomalous direction of eruption of the impacted tooth itself or a neighbouring tooth acting as an obstacle. For example, the upper canine, in its germ phase, is located very high, deep in the maxilla and close to the orbit, and is directed to its corresponding place in the arch very late, when the adjacent teeth have already erupted. Supernumerary teeth acting as a barrier, bone density and chronic non-infectious inflammation also play a role. Another very frequent cause is the negative bone-tooth discrepancy which results in a lack of space in the dental arch due to mandibular or maxillary micrognathism, anomalies in the size and shape of the teeth, presence of supernumerary teeth, among others. Pathologically inserted upper labial frenulum, loss of primary teeth due to caries, persistence of primary teeth, cystic and tumour disease can be causes of retention. A root cyst of a primary tooth with necrotic pulp can cause retention of the successor permanent tooth. The existence of a dentigerous and follicular cyst can represent an obstacle to the eruption of the affected permanent tooth. These cysts are relatively common; they engulf the crown of the tooth and insert into the neck of the tooth. The roots of the tooth are outside the cystic sac. The developmental dentigerous cyst is one of the most frequent and can be the cause of inclusion, impaction or tooth retention, more predominant in permanent teeth and supernumerary teeth than in deciduous teeth. Odontomas and other odontogenic and non-odontogenic tumours are also frequent. Seventy-five percent of odontomas are diagnosed between the first and second decades of life due to a delay in permanent tooth eruption, as they are asymptomatic and there is no significant gender predilection. Another local cause is infectious disease. It has been described and observed in clinical practice that in the area of retained teeth, especially third molars, which suffer local infections, fibrosis is caused in the mucosa covering the tooth that is about to erupt in the healing process that occurs when the infection is resolved, especially in pericoronaritis, which prevents the eruption of the dental organ. On the other hand, there is dental alveolar trauma, since in the area of the buccal mucosa that has suffered severe trauma (dental alveolar fracture, fracture of the mandible or maxilla), a different bone density is caused, as well as a change in the morphology of the mucosa that can make it more fibrous, preventing the eruption of the tooth that is about to erupt. In cases of patients who have lost molars and are rehabilitated without an X-ray, the repetitive trauma to the mucosa causes a change in the morphology of the mucosa that makes it more fibrous and prevents the eruption of the tooth. ,[2328] , [29]

Reduced masticatory function, occlusal and interproximal abrasion due to edge-to-edge occlusion and the consequences of orthodontic treatment also cause tooth retention. In addition, in cases of premature extraction of a deciduous tooth, when the germ of the permanent tooth is distant from its eruption site in the dental arch, the alveolus may be closed by a bony bridge, which, due to its density, acts as an obstacle that the permanent tooth cannot overcome. In these cases, both the bone and the gum heal. In the case of the gingiva, it becomes a dense, sclerotic tissue due to occlusal and masticatory trauma over time.[30] , [31]

Systemic factors:

General causes are systemic diseases including physiological delay of eruption such as irradiation, endocrine disorders, metabolic disorders, hereditary conditions, Gardner syndrome, cleidocranial dysostosis, hereditary ectodermal polydysplasia, fibrous dysplasias and osteopetrosis or Albers-Schonberg disease.[32]

There are also congenital factors due to maternal pathologies during pregnancy, such as: trauma, maternal diet, chicken pox, other viruses and alterations in maternal metabolism. Race mixing is also considered as a cause of eruption alteration, it has been proved that in homogeneous racial groups, the frequency of malocclusion is low and:where there has been racial mixing, jaw size discrepancy and disorders are significantly greater, some studies show that there may be a dominance of "effect" over "excess", in terms of the size of the components of the stomatognathic apparatus, as a result of racial mixing; These studies are consistent with studies by anthropologists indicating that the jaws are shrinking in size, thus there is an increased frequency of included third molars or congenital lack of some teeth, as well as a tendency towards retrognathism as we move up the phylogenetic scale. Other systemic causes are some forms of anaemia, syphilis, tuberculosis, malnutrition, rickets, scurvy, BeriBeri. They often influence the course of tooth eruption, premature exfoliation and prolonged retention of teeth. Among endocrine dysfunctions, the most characteristic for tooth retention are subclinical hypothyroidism, premature sexual or gonadal development and hormonal iatrogenesis.[33]

Rare conditions include cleidocranial dysostosis or dysplasia, a rare autosomal dominant condition, characterised by: cranial widening at the expense of the frontal and parietal bones, with very wide fontanels that take years to close, mild atrophy of the upper facial mass and exophthalmos, multiple dental anomalies, such as retardation of both dentitions and dental absences and inclusions, sometimes multiple. Also hypoplasia or aplasia of both clavicles, spina bifida and limb malformations, oxycephaly, tower skull caused by rapid fusion of multiple sutures, progeria or premature blindness, achondroplasia and cleft lip, maxilla and palate. Crouzon syndrome, characterised by premature closure of the cranial sutures, is also commonly found. Prominent forehead, prognathism, exophthalmos, with possible dislocation of the eyeball, beaked nose, shortened upper lip and low-set but normal morphology of the pinnae are observed.[34]

Alterations of systemic aetiology have generalised manifestation on the eruption, single or few teeth alterations usually have local causalities.[35]

Diagnosis of tooth retention

It is the responsibility of the general dentist to achieve an early diagnosis of this pathology, preferably before the age of 9 and up to 12 years, with the main objective of preventing retention.[30]

The diagnosis of this entity is made on the basis of the clinical picture, supported by views and radiographic images. It is necessary to carry out a detailed interrogation to look for possible causes of retention, framing them into local and systemic causes, and to perform a thorough physical examination. In the extrabuccal examination, the angle of the mandible can be examined and the prominence of the bone at this level can be seen; in the scalp, alopecia aereata can sometimes be observed and in the region of the middle third of the face, the protrusion of the eyeball that can be seen in some patients with dentigerous cysts associated with retained teeth and in relation to the maxillary sinus. An adequate examination of the tissues surrounding the area of retention, morphological characteristics of the gingiva, presence of local infections, scar flanges, pericoronal caps, lacerations in the mucosa of the cheek, haematomas, change of colour of the mucosa covering the tooth, etc. should be carried out. In the intraoral physical examination the following are most important: absence of the tooth past the age of eruption, increase in volume, persistence of the temporary tooth, pain, malocclusion, inclination or irregular positioning of adjacent teeth, eruption cysts, pericoronaritis (mild, moderate, severe), limitation of oral opening.[36]

It is essential to complement the clinical examination with a radiographic study in order to make an accurate diagnosis. The diagnosis that a radiograph allows is necessary, as different characteristics and specific areas can be assessed. Therefore, it is considered an examination of medical-legal value, and essential in the diagnosis of any type of disease or clinical alteration. Although simple radiographs are not considered conclusive in a diagnosis, as they must be carried out using the correct technique, they are of great importance in providing information to the dentist. , ,[373839]

Radiographic study

The radiographic study can be aided by intraoral views such as periapical radiography, the parallax or Clark technique and occlusal radiography. Extraoral views such as panoramic radiography, lateral oblique mandibular radiography and computerised axial tomography (CT) are also used. The latter provides more information of the canine in all three planes of space. CT scans are a non-invasive, high-cost examination.[40] , [41]

Cone Beam computed tomography is a method that has advanced the field of dental radiology, since it achieves very high resolution computed tomography (3D) images of the craniofacial space. It can provide images of muscles, bones, organs, blood vessels, fat, revealing a structure in several dimensions and with a wide visual acuity. 42,43

The radiographic study makes it possible to determine the depth of the impaction measured in relation to the occlusal plane, the direction and angle of inclination of the tooth compared to the axial axis of the adjacent erupted tooth, the length, shape, direction and number of roots. Other aspects that can be visualised are the shape and size of the crown, the periodontal ligament space, the close relationship to structures whose preservation is essential, especially the lower dental canal or the maxillary sinus, the presence of radiolucent lesions in relation to the included tooth and the possibility of ankylosis or hypercementosis.[33]

Classifications of tooth retention

In the literature we can find various classifications to describe the position of retained teeth, the most commonly used are those of Winter and Pell and Gregory, which focus on third molars, Trujillo Fandiño, which describes the position of retained incisors, canines and premolars, Field and Ackerman, which refers to retained incisors and canines, and Ugalde, which deals with canines and premolars.[44]

Trujillo[45] classifies the location of the crown of the retained tooth organ in relation to the cervical, middle and apical root thirds of the adjacent teeth and establishes 5 mm for each root third, as follows:

- Position I: When the crown or the major part of the crown is at the level of the cervical third of the root of the adjacent teeth in dentate jaws. And in the space between the alveolar ridge up to 5 mm from the alveolar ridge in the maxilla equivalent to the cervical third.
- Position II: When the crown or most of the crown is at the level of the middle third of the roots of the adjacent teeth in dentate jaws. And in the space between 5 and 10 mm from the alveolar ridge of the jaws, equivalent to the middle third.
- Position III: When the crown or most of it is located at the level of the apical third of the root of the adjacent teeth in dentate jaws. And in a space 10 mm or more from the alveolar ridge of the jaws.
- On the other hand, Echegaray26 describes Field and Ackerman's classification which states:
- Vestibular position: the crown is attached to the incisors or to the crown above the apices of the incisors.
- Palatal/Lingual position: represented by the crown being close to the surface and in correlation with the roots of the incisors.
- Mid position: the crown is placed between the roots of the lateral incisor and the first premolar with the crown above the roots of these teeth towards the vestibular and the root towards the palatal or vice versa.

Ugalde[46] in 2001 formulated a classification of canines and premolars by means of a series of parameters, such as angulation, depth, root formation:

Angulation

Analyses the angulation of the impacted canine in relation to the occlusal plane.

- Horizontal: when the longitudinal axis of the canine in relation to the occlusal plane has an angulation between 0 and 30 degrees.

- Mesioangular: when the angulation shall be from 31 to 60 degrees.
- Vertical: angulation of the longitudinal axis of the canine and occlusal plane between 61-90 degrees.
- Distoangular: the angulation corresponds to 91 degrees and upwards.
- Inverted: crown to apical Depth

Measured from the occlusal plane to the cusp of the retained canine thus obtaining:

- Surface retention no more than 5mm.
- Moderate retention up to 10mm.
- Retentiondepthmiddlemorethan10mm Root formation

According to their root development they can be:

- In training.
- Full training.
- Dislacerated

Consequences of tooth retention

In the childhood stage it is considered essential that parents are correctly informed about the period of exfoliation, as they will be aware of how long deciduous teeth should remain in the mouth, they will be able to detect any anomaly in this process and thus be able to go to the specialists immediately and intercept the problem in time. In many cases, tooth retention syndrome is already noticeable during adolescence, as the patient tends to recognise the anomaly due to aesthetics or associated symptoms. Early diagnosis will be vital for the problem, as it will detect permanent teeth that have deviated from their normal course or eruption pathway or have been retained because of a primary tooth that has not been exfoliated. By intervening in time, other alterations such as malocclusion, dental ankylosis can be avoided and the prognosis will be more beneficial as well as the treatment. Retention of permanent teeth is a fairly recurrent condition in children and adolescents and sometimes the prognosis is difficult for the orthodontist. There is considerable parental concern about the lack of early diagnosis, also due to late identification of the main risk factors, as well as the aesthetic, occlusal, psychosocial consequences and uncertainty in the application of an adequate technique that provides a high margin of safety in terms of the integrity of neighbouring teeth and favourable results.[10], [47]

Retained teeth, like any other tooth, can cause disorders of mechanical, infectious, nervous and tumoural origin. Among those of mechanical origin we have: lingual or labial malposition of the retained tooth, migration of the neighbouring tooth and loss of arch length, internal resorption, internal dentigerous formation, external root resorption of the retained canine, as well as of the neighbouring teeth. On the other hand referred pain, pericoronaritis and localised periodontal disease in adjacent teeth are due to disorders of infectious origin. From a nervous point of view, nerve fibre compressions can occur and cause neuralgia. Tumour disorders are mostly due to chronic infection of the pericoronary sac, apical infection, periodontitis and the development of cysts of the dental follicle. These disorders include granulomas, root cysts, odentigerous follicular cysts, ameloblastomas and malignant tumours.[20]

A patient with retention or delay of the canine teeth may be the result of an endocrine or thyroid disorder, gingival fibrosis, or others such as malposition of the teeth prior to their eruption, or also due to a lack of space in the dental arch.[48]

Restrepo and Mariaca[49], point out that: "Canines are very important for the oral health of people, as well as for their facial aesthetics, in addition to the functions they have in occlusion, which is why periodontal treatment is usually applied when they are retained. Among the sequelae we can highlight: eruptive alterations that affect the aesthetics of the person, loss of contour of the maxilla, reabsorption of the lateral incisor, generalised pain at the mandibular level, deviation of the midline, nervous system disorders, mesialisation of the posterior area causing loss of the affected space, dental transmigration, giroversion and inclination of the lateral incisor from the affected position, among others".

Therapeutic options for impacted teeth

In order to choose the appropriate therapeutic management for each patient, a careful evaluation of the developmental stage of the dentition and assessment of risk agents is essential, as treatment is highly dependent on factors such as age, tooth position and the patient's systemic condition. Treatment of impacted teeth is necessary in order to avoid dental sequelae at a later age. For this reason, early diagnosis is recommended and the general dentist should carry out an exhaustive evaluation of the patient, including a multidisciplinary study.[27]

Among the treatments used is abstention, which is decided when there is a general contraindication to surgical intervention, because the manipulation of the included tooth can lead to complications such as the loss of other healthy teeth, or when the tooth is totally included in the maxilla, with a minimum of 2 mm of bone around its perimeter. Some authors call it a "mute" inclusion because of the small percentage of alteration it produces. If this variant is highlighted, it is advisable to monitor the patient regularly, both clinically and radiographically, in order to minimise the risk of future disorders.[50]

Tooth extraction is indicated when the retained tooth causes pain or discomfort to the patient, when it causes infections or pockets and resorption of bone and the root of a neighbouring tooth. This therapeutic option is also chosen when it causes malocclusions, such as crowding, migrations, rotations, collapse of the dental arch, etc., when it is associated with a cyst or tumour, in patients who are going to undergo ionising radiation or orthognathic surgery, or in cases where the retained tooth is included in the focus of a fracture of the jaw, as it turns it into an open fracture, as well as to avoid infections in the focus of the fracture.[51]

When the included tooth has aesthetic and functional value, manoeuvres or procedures must be carried out to place it in the dental arch, which must not be dangerous or jeopardise the vitality of the tooth or the adjacent teeth. Treatment must be imposed early on to prevent the teeth from deviating and erupting in an anomalous position. The following surgical techniques are used for this purpose:

- Conductive alveolotomy: As its name indicates, no type of oral tissue is excised. It is widely used in moderate and mild inclusions, which can be diagnosed by observing a bulge near the place where the tooth should occupy and which corresponds to the crown of the tooth. In this case, an apical repositioning flap is performed, leaving the crown of the included tooth uncovered, repositioning the flap towards the apical and suturing it higher than its initial position.

- Conductive Alveolectomy: This technique is indicated for moderate and mild inclusions. It involves a gingivectomy or simple excision of the gum covering the included tooth, normally this gum can be fibrous and therefore becomes an obstacle to the normal eruption of the tooth, a collar of gum is left around the tooth, approximately 3 mm, then surgical cement is placed to prevent the wound from closing.

- Tooth transplantation: Reimplantation, Transplantation (autologous, homologous, heterologous), implant, relocation. [23]

Orthodontic-surgical methods are procedures that combine surgery and orthodontics, with the aim of placing a tooth in its normal position. Each speciality in the treatment plays a different role but the final objective is the same, the surgery must be able to achieve the discovery of the tooth and its correct visualisation and allow the orthodontist to place the necessary elements for the traction. Another variant is dental fenestration and orthodontic treatment used in severe inclusions, when the longitudinal axis of the included tooth is parallel to the longitudinal axis of the neighbouring tooth, mucosa and bone is removed around the included tooth, with the aim of freeing and visualising the crown and then being able to place a obracket button. This attachment or traction device is used to activate the tooth, which is then placed in its correct position in the dental arch. The loop technique can also be used as a means of traction. This consists of passing a stainless steel wire around the neck of the tooth, twisting it carefully to prevent it from exceeding the anatomical constriction of the neck of the canine. Other means can be: pre-formed orthodontic band, stainless steel crown, threaded or cemented pin, metal ligature placed through a hole made in the crown of the impacted tooth, cemented button and others. In the case of severe inclusions, fenestration, repositioning and orthodontic treatment is used when the longitudinal axis of the included tooth is slightly deviated with respect to the longitudinal axis of the neighbouring tooth; First, fenestration is carried out, i.e. the removal of mucosa and bone around the tooth and a slight movement is added to the tooth with the aim of repositioning it, i.e. correcting the deviation of its longitudinal axis. This small movement must be very careful and moderate, carried out with slight movements executed with elevators. It should be pointed out that the indispensable requirement for repositioning is when the tooth has approximately 2/3 of the root formed. It is not recommended when the included tooth already has a fully developed root. As a means of traction, those described above for fenestration and surgical treatment can be used.[52]

Prevention of tooth retention

Prevention consists of a set of actions carried out by professionals, technicians and the population itself, in order to avoid the installation of a certain disease in individuals and groups or during the different stages of the disease, with the aim of limiting complications and sequelae. The study of the factors involved in the course of diseases and their prevention is a fundamental part of the health professional's work. In the case of a non-communicable disease such as dental impaction, prevention must also be aimed at avoiding complications or sequelae. For this purpose, early diagnosis and timely treatment are available, so that actions at the secondary level are carried out. These are generally carried out by the general stomatologist and the orthodontist, sometimes it is not thought that this action is also preventive, but it is.[53] , 54, 55

Interceptive orthodontics is closely related to this level of prevention, early transverse expansions in cases of micrognathism and indications for tooth extractions based on sound criteria are very clear options. The implementation of a change in the habits of the patient and his family together with an adequate medical control before the development of a specific pathology should be the basis of the health system, since this would prevent the disease, subsequent complications and morbidity and mortality, which would benefit not only the patient and his family but also the state, since the medical and economic resources now available can be used more effectively in people whose pathologies cannot be prevented.[56]

Authors such as Couto et al.[57] , analysed the prevalence and factors associated with malocclusions in preschool children in the town of Aiquara in Brazil, where deleterious oral habits (tete, onychophagia and digital suction) and diseases such as dental caries are associated with malocclusions, emphasising the need for ongoing educational activities.

A study conducted in Chennai, India, addressing the level of awareness and knowledge of parents about malocclusion in their children, showed a lack of awareness of the importance of maintenance of primary teeth to prevent irregular tooth arrangement in a child. Other research in central India showed a high proportion of children requiring preventive and interceptive treatment.[58] , [59]

In general, there is insufficient information about activities for the prevention of permanent canine retention in infants and adolescents, so a group of actions are suggested that could be taken into account. These include the development of a system of general health promotion and prevention actions in the community, the implementation of educational activities aimed at parents and relatives of patients with the anomaly about the treatment process and the infant and adolescent population in general. Also the application of an instrument for the early classification of groups vulnerable to the anomaly and the practical application of preventive and interceptive orthodontics. Risk factors such as premature extraction of primary teeth, transverse micrognathism, persistence of primary teeth, deforming habits, among others, must be controlled. It is essential to carry out radiographic studies in the high-risk adolescent population in order to achieve an early imaging diagnosis and evaluate possible treatment, as well as to establish an algorithm for comprehensive multidisciplinary care of the paediatric population with retained maxillary canines, prioritising interconsultations with specialists in maxillofacial surgery, orthodontics and periodontology.[30]

METHODOLOGICAL DESIGN

A descriptive, cross-sectional study was carried out in the orthodontic clinic of the Manuel Piti Fajardo Polyclinic, during the period from January 2023 to March 2024. The population consisted of all students between 8 and 19 years of age from the schools who attended the clinic and were diagnosed with retained permanent anterior teeth, 67 cases of which were counted. Sampling was not used as the total population was used.

Methods, techniques and instruments to be used:

The research used a combination of theoretical, empirical and statistical methods for data collection, processing and evaluation.

<u>Theoretical methods:</u>

> The historical-logical study facilitated a study of the logical historical evolution of the behaviour of tooth retention, as well as to determine the essence and trends of the trajectory of this anomaly. It made it possible to visualise the stepwise continuity of the research.

> The analytical-synthetic approach was used in the systematisation of scientific and pedagogical texts, normative documents, as well as in the establishment of relations, interactions and generalisations of the research. It was used throughout the research.

> The inductive-deductive approach made it possible to process the empirical information obtained and to move from a knowledge of particular cases to a more general one and vice versa. <u>Empirical methods:</u>

> Observation: this was used to obtain the variables of interest for this research, as well as to assess the radiographs that were indicated.

> Form: This was used to collect the variables of interest for this research.

<u>Statistical methods:</u>

Descriptive statistics and non-parametric inferential statistics (chi-square) were applied in the research.

The data were entered into an automated database using Microsoft Office 2010, Excel

2010, running on Windows on a personal microcomputer. Frequency distributions and crosstabulations of variables according to their different attributes were obtained from the database. Descriptive statistical techniques were applied and tables were drawn up in which the values of the attributes of the variables were expressed in absolute frequencies and percentages.

The main variables used were: age, sex, retained tooth according to the order in the arch, location of the retained incisor or canine, position, cause of retention and treatment of choice.

Operationalisation and conceptualisation of variables:

VARIABLES	CLASSIFICATION	DEFINITION OF THE VARIABLE	GRADING SCALE
Sex	Qualitative nominal dichotomous	According to the biological sex to which they belong.	Female Male
Age	Continuous quantitative	Years completed according to IQ	8,9,10,11,12,13,14,15,16,17,18,19
Retained tooth	Qualitative Nominal Qualitative Polytomous	According to the anatomy and order of the dental arch	Upper central incisor Upper lateral incisor Lower central incisor Lower lateral incisor Upper canines Lower canines

Location of the impacted incisor or canine	Qualitative Nominal Qualitative Polytomous	Depending on the location of the tooth in question in the arch, and whether it is unilateral or bilateral	Upper right Upper left Lower right Lower left Bilateral upper Bilateral lower
Position of the retained tooth	Qualitative Nominal Qualitative Polytomous	Depending on the position of the retained tooth	Vestibular Lingual/Palatine Medium
Cause of retention	Qualitative Nominal Qualitative Polytomous	Depending on the cause of tooth retention	Premises: Irregular tooth position or pressure from an adjacent tooth (Supernumerary teeth and direction)
			Anomalous eruption of the tooth itself) Bone density Persistence of the storm Gingival fibrosis Chronic non-infectious inflammation Negative tooth-bone discrepancy Cystic and tumour disease: Root cyst of a primary tooth, dentigerous cyst, odontoma Infectious disease Alveolar tooth trauma Systemic: Prenatal causes: hereditary and genetic, congenital mixed-race Postnatal causes: anaemia, syphilis, tuberculosis, malnutrition, scurvy, Beri Beri, endocrine dysfunction, hypothyroidism, early sexual development Rare conditions: Cleidocranial dysplasia, Crouzon Syndrome

Treatment of choice	Qualitative Nominal Qualitative Polytomous	Depending on the treatment variant chosen	Abstention Tooth extraction Orthodontic treatment Orthodontic-surgical treatment

Processing, analysis of information and techniques to be used.

The results were processed by manual methods and the data obtained were entered into a database using the Statistical Package for the Social Sciences (SPSS), version 15.0 for Windows. Microsoft Office 2010, Excel 2010, was used for this purpose. Frequency distributions and crosstabulations of variables according to their different attributes were obtained from the database. Descriptive statistics techniques were applied, and tables were drawn up in which the values of the attributes of the variables were expressed in absolute frequencies and percentages. In non-parametric inferential statistics, the non-parametric Chi-square test (X2) was used, as well as the significance test associated with it. According to the p-value, it was classified as follows: Significant: If $p<0.05$.

Not significant: If $p>= 0.05$

Procedures:

1. First Stage: Authorisation to carry out the research was requested from the centre's management (Annex 1), explaining the purpose of the research, as well as the procedures that would be carried out, all under the commitment to medical ethics.

2. Second Stage: The clinical examination of the patients who gave their informed consent (Appendix 2) was carried out at the consultation, as well as the indication and interpretation of periapical X-rays, taking into account an observation guide (Appendix 3) to obtain the variables of interest for the research. This information was collected on a form previously designed for this purpose (Appendix 4).

3. Stage Three: All the information was entered into a computerised database for statistical processing and subsequent presentation in tables.

Ethical Aspects

The study was carried out based on international ethical standards for experimental and biomedical research with humans (Nuremberg Code, Declaration of Helsinki I and II, United Nations Principles of Medical Ethics, CIOMS Ethical Standards, Universal Declaration on the Human Genome and Human Rights) and National Ethical Standards, such as the principles of Medical Ethics and Ethical Standards of Good Practice in Human Experimentation. These standards were taken into account from the design of the research project, with strict compliance throughout the study process and culminating in the presentation of the results.

On this basis, informed consent was obtained from the management of the "Manuel Piti Fajardo" Polyclinic (Appendix 1) after explaining what the research would consist of.

The information obtained was used only for this purpose, and it was explained to each patient what the study would consist of, making it clear that it would not involve any harm to their health. The X-rays taken would be completely safe for the students. In this respect, we drew up a model of informed consent that was signed by each patient or their parent or guardian (Appendix 2), within the basic principles to be taken into account, in order to satisfy the moral, ethical and legal requirements in research with human beings and not to violate the bioethical principles of beneficence, non-maleficence, autonomy and justice.

RESULTS

Table 1. Distribution according to age and sex of retained permanent anterior teeth. Manuel Piti Fajardo Polyclinic. Santo Domingo (January 2023 to March 2024)

Sex	Age			
	FA	%	Media	esviació n standard
Female	26	38.8	12,1	2,63
Male	41	61.2	11,4	2,44
Total	67	100		

Source: Form

The table groups the students with retained permanent anterior teeth according to sex. Forty-one males were found to be affected with this anomaly in the study population, representing 61.2% of the total population. In the female sex, 26 patients were found to be affected, representing 38.8% of the total. It is worth noting the superiority of the male sex in this result. With regard to age, the mean age of the females was 12.1 years, with a standard deviation of 2.63. In males, the mean age was 11.4 years with a deviation of 2.44 years.

Table 2. Distribution according to location of retained permanent anterior teeth

Group		FA	%
Incisors	Upper right lateral incisor	2	3,0
	Upper left central incisor	6	9,0
	Lower left lateral incisor	7	10,4
	Upper right central incisor	3	4,5
	Lower left central incisor	2	3,0
	Right upper central incisor and Left upper central incisor	4	6,0
Canines	Lower right canine	13	19,4
	Lower left canine	11	16,4
	Upper right canine	7	10,4
	Upper left canine	12	17,9
Total		67	100,0

Source: Form

The table shows that canines were the teeth most affected by tooth retention, and as a general rule, most patients had only one retained tooth. There was the highest incidence of retained lower right canine with a total of 13 patients for 19.4% of the total, followed by the upper left canine with 12 patients representing 17.9%. This was followed by the lower left canine with 11 patients representing 16.4% and the upper right canine with 7 patients for 10.4% of the total. The least affected teeth in the study population were the upper right lateral incisor and the lower left central incisor with 2 patients each, corresponding to 3% respectively.

Table 3. Distribution of patients with retained anterior and permanent anterior teeth according to position

Position	FA	%
Vestibular	51	76,1
Palatine	4	6,0
Lingual	11	16,4
Medium	1	1,5
Total	67	100,0

Source: Form

The table shows a predominance of the vestibular position with a total of 51 patients with teeth retained in this position, which represented 76.1% of the total, followed by the lingual position with 11 patients for 16.4%, the palatal position with 4 for 6% and the least frequent was the mid position with only 1 student with a tooth retained in this position, which corresponded to 1.5% of the total.

Table 4. Determination of the causes of tooth retention in the study population.

	Causes	FA	%
Premises	Gingival fibrosis	8	11,9
	Persistence of the storm	22	32,8
	Negative H-D discrepancy	20	29,9
	Odontoma	6	9,0
	Supernumerary	5	7,5
	Malposition of the canine	6	9,0
	Total	67	100,0

Source: Form

The table shows that the most frequent causes of tooth retention in the study population were local. Temporal impaction was predominant with 22 patients, representing 32.8 % of the total, and negative bone-tooth discrepancy with 20 patients, representing 29.9 % of the total. This was followed by gingival fibrosis with 8 patients, corresponding to 11.9 %, odontoma and canine malposition with 6 patients each, representing 9 % of the total. Lastly, the presence of supernumerary teeth was found with 5 affected children, representing 7.5 % of the population. No systemic causes of tooth retention were found.

Table 5. Determination of treatment for dental retention in the patients under study

Treatments	FA	%
Abstention	8	11,9
Tooth extraction	25	37,3
Orthodontic treatment	20	29,9
Treatment Surgical orthodontics	14	20,9
Total	67	100,0

Source: Form

The table shows the predominance of the therapeutic variant of tooth extraction in

25 patients, for 37.3 % of the total, as the retained teeth caused malocclusions or odontomas in some cases, followed by orthodontic treatment in 20 students for 29.9 %. This was followed by orthodontic-surgical treatment in 14 patients (20.9% of the total) and the least frequent treatment was abstention, which was carried out in 8 patients (11.9%) because of general contraindications to surgical intervention or because manipulation of the impacted tooth could lead to complications such as loss of other healthy teeth. Therapeutic abstention is not advisable because of the risk of infection, cysts and root resorption in adjacent teeth.

Table 6. Position of the tooth retention according to sex

Position /sex	Female		Male		Total	
	No	%	N o	%	No	%
vestibular	18	69.2	33	80.5	51	76.1
Palatine	2	7.7	2	4.9	4	6.0
Lingual	5	19.2	6	14.6	11	16.4
Medium	1	3.8	0	0	1	1.5
Total	26	100	41	100	67	100

Source: Form

F=2,396;=0,565>0,050

The table shows that in the female sex the vestibular position of the retained teeth predominated (69.2%) as did the male sex with 33 patients (80.5% of the total of the male sex). The median position was only seen in one female patient, which represented 3.8% of the total. The Fisher's F test showed that p> 0.050, a non-significant result, so that the position in which the event is detected does not depend on sex.

Table 7. Treatment of the retained components by gender

Treatment/sex	Female		Male		Total	
	N o	%	N o	%	No	%
Abstention	3	11.5	5	12.2	8	12
Tooth extraction	9	34.6	16	39.0	25	37.3
Orthodontic treatment	7	26.9	13	31.7	20	29.9
Surgical orthodontic treatment	7	26.9	7	17.1	14	20.9
Total	26	100	41	100	67	100

Source: Form

F=1,044 ;=0,814>0,050

The table shows that in the female sex the most frequently indicated treatment was tooth extraction, with 9 patients for 34.6% of the total number of girls, as well as in the male sex with a total of 16 patients, representing 39% of the male sex. The treatment that was applied the least was abstention, with 3 patients in the female sex for 11.5% and 5 patients in the male sex representing 12.2%, as the conditions for deciding on this therapeutic variant were less frequent. When statistical processing was carried out, it was found that $p > 0.050$, a non-significant result, so there is no dependency relationship between the treatment of the retained tooth and sex.

DISCUSSION OF THE RESULTS

In the research carried out, a prevalence of the male sex affected by retained permanent anterior teeth was observed. This coincides with Román[60] who in his study: "Prevalence of retained canines in the dental office", in Ecuador, states that 55% of the patients with retained teeth were men and 45% were women. With similar results, Segura[20] in his graduate work entitled: "Prevalence of retained anterior teeth in paediatric patients", at the University of Guayaquil, highlights a slight predominance of the male sex.

However, most of the studies highlight a higher incidence in the female sex. Such is the case of Mendoza et al.[61] , who report a prevalence of 61.2% and 38.8% of affected cases in the state of Hidalgo, respectively. They also differ from the results of the author, Pichel et al.[48] , in their research to identify dental retention in patients at the José Martí Polyclinic in Cuba, in 122 children of both sexes, in which they determine that females are the most affected (62.2%).

As a researcher, I believe that most studies conclude that boys are less affected by tooth retention, as their jaws are larger than those of girls, so there is more space available for dental alignment. On the other hand, the eruption cycle begins earlier in females than in males, which is related to hormonal factors and if there is any type of alteration during this period it is detectable earlier in females. Furthermore, the prevalence of the female sex is also frequent in the different orthodontic studies concerned with aesthetics, although both sexes currently attend in equal proportions.

It is common to find dental impaction with increasing age, as it is necessary to assess the age of sprouting and chronological age for diagnosis. [62]

In this study, the mean age of females was about one year higher than that of males. It was not possible to make comparisons with other authors. I believe that this is due to the fact that the data collection was different in the age group 8 to 11 years, where retained incisors are more frequent, while in patients aged 12 to 19 years, it is common to find retained canines.

In the present investigation, the most frequently retained permanent anterior teeth were the canines, both upper and lower. This result is similar to that described by Pichel et al.[48] , who found that the most frequently retained teeth were the canines (62.2%) and the least represented were the incisors (6.5%).

According to Perez[63] , in his thesis entitled: "Causes and incidences of retention in permanent canines", developed in Ecuador, the right upper canine is the most frequently retained, followed by the left upper canine. Bilateral retention of the upper canines is also very frequent. Among the lower canines, retention of the right lower canine is more frequent. The author agrees with this result, as this was the most frequently retained tooth in the study population.

Segura[20] also provides a similar result in his study to determine the prevalence of impacted anterior teeth in paediatric patients, in which he states that canines are the teeth most affected by this anomaly.

They differ from the research findings of Fundora et al.[2] , in their publication entitled: "Characterisation of patients operated on for dental retention in Pinar del Río, 2017-2018", which reveal that the most frequently retained teeth are the third molars with 60.7%, followed by the canines with 52.4% in terms of incidence; likewise, Suárez[64] , in his study: "Prevalence of retained dental pieces in patients aged 15 to 60 years seen at the Cero Huánuco 2018 radiology centre",mentions in order of frequency that the upper third molars top the list with 41.1%, followed by the upper canine with a figure of 23.67%.

In my opinion, the canines were the most affected teeth, since, first of all, this study only dealt with the anterior sector. It is important to note that they are among the last teeth to erupt in the maxilla, so they often present problems for proper placement. Furthermore, they are located in a real anatomical and ontogenetic crossroads and their germ occupies a very high position from which they must carry out their eruptive movements in an orientation that is not always favourable. In the case of the lower canines, it was common for them to be retained, fundamentally due to prolonged retention of the temporomandibular molars and the lack of space in the dental arch.

With regard to the position of the retention, a greater predominance of retained teeth was found in the vestibular position, and the least frequent was the medial position. In this last aspect, the researcher agrees with Echegaray[26] and Miranda et al.[50] , however we differ with these authors regarding the most prevalent position, as they highlight a predominance of retained teeth in the palatal position in 60 % of the cases, while the vestibular position has a proportion of 30 %, and the remaining 10 % are in the mid position. The author also disagrees with Mendoza et al.[61] , who point out that "the prevalence in terms of location is 85% in the palatal position, 13% in the middle and 1.6% in the vestibular position"; as does Ayala et al.[65] , in their publication: "Dental eruption and its influencing factors", in which they express a greater predominance of teeth retained in the palatal position.

I consider that retention of teeth in the vestibular area is associated with space problems, while palatal impaction is related to alterations in the trajectory, both of which are scientifically supported. The path that the canine has to follow, for example, from the point where its germ is formed until it emerges in the arch, is much longer and more complex than that followed by any other tooth, which would explain any deviation in eruptive guidance. The results obtained pointed more to retention in the vestibular position, as it was very common to find that patients had very little space for proper dental alignment.

In relation to the causes of dental retention, the predominant cause was the persistence of the primary tooth, followed by the negative bone-tooth discrepancy, and odontoma was among the least frequent. Similar results were obtained by Echegaray[26] , in Ecuador, in his degree thesis entitled: "Etiological factors that cause retention of permanent canines". where he determined that the main causes of retention are: negative bone-tooth discrepancy, prolonged maintenance of primary teeth, followed by the premature loss of these teeth caused by the extraction or premature loss of the primary tooth, which in the long term can lead to a reduction in the size of the arch and the presence of odontomas, cysts or tumours.

The researcher also agrees with Quevedo[24] , who in her publication "Causas locales de caninos permanentes retenidos en pacientes de la Clínica Estomatológica René Guzmán Pérez de Calixto García", Holguín, indicates that the greatest prevalence of retained anterior teeth is due to the presence of a small arch in relation to the size of the teeth. On the other hand, it is evident that there is consensus with Segura[20] , who states that the retention of anterior teeth may be due to anterior crowding, due to the absence or reduced space that does not allow the permanent tooth to be lodged.

In a degree thesis developed in Bolivia by Quisbert[66] , entitled: "Aetiology and incidence in the retention of permanent canines", it is stated that 5% of the cases of patients with retention of permanent anterior teeth, present odontoma or tumour, which constitutes the least cause of retention in that study, which is similar to the current research, where it was one of the least representative factors.

However, it differs with the findings of Echegaray[26] , who considers that in addition to local causes, it is important to consider alterations in the embryological stage and systemic factors such as physiological delay of eruption due to a mismatch between physiological and chronological age.

Another study that does not agree with the results obtained is the one carried out in Peru, entitled: "Frequency of retained canines in patients aged 14 to 20 years", which suggests that one of the causes is genetic as well as hereditary or generic factors as sources of this dental anomaly.[67]

Pichel et al.[48] , who add that dental retention is due to dental eruptive alterations, associated with phylogenetic factors, endocrine disorders, others are closely related to metabolism, congenital ectodermal polydysplasia and osteoporosis, also differ from what was observed in the population under study.

As a researcher, I believe that there was a greater prevalence of local causes, mainly the persistence of the rainstorm beyond the time of its exfoliation, since two years passed during which the world's population was affected by COVID 19, during which time most services were paralysed and parents stopped taking their children to dental clinics. As the pandemic was brought under control, parents' lack of interest in this anomaly prevailed, so it went unnoticed and early and timely diagnosis in primary care was not possible.

The predominant treatment variant according to this study was tooth extraction, followed by orthodontic treatment. This coincides with Quintana et al.68 and Díaz 69, in their studies carried out in Artemisa (Cuba) and Peru respectively, who highlight tooth extraction as the most frequently implemented treatment. It also agrees with Rodríguez et al13 , who in their study entitled: "Multidisciplinary treatment of retained teeth in Granma, indicate "that extraction is one of the most commonly used treatments in cases of retained teeth that do not present major symptoms, followed by orthodontic treatment, depending on the precise diagnosis".

The author differs with Corrales[70] in her research "Tratamiento ortodóncico- quirúrgico de caninos retenidos en paciente de 14 años", in Pinar del Rio and with Carballido[40] , in her publication in Madrid: "Diagnóstico de canino incluido", both of which determine a predominance of orthodontic-surgical treatment.

I consider that tooth extraction was the most commonly implemented treatment, as the retained teeth in many cases caused malocclusions such as crowding, rotations, versions, migrations, collapse of the dental arch, among other anomalies. In some patients they were also associated with odontomas, which was the immediate course of action. Other reasons for deciding to extract teeth, in addition to the occlusal complications mentioned above, were the aesthetic and psychosocial consequences for the students who made up the study population.

On analysing the possible association between sex and the position of tooth retention, it was concluded that there was no dependence, as both females and males were more likely to retain teeth in the vestibular position. No studies were found that coincided with the results obtained; however, they disagree with the author, Segura[20] and Cornejo[71] who state that retention is more common in the female sex in the palatal position. As a researcher, I believe that teeth retained in the vestibular position were the most common in both sexes, without distinction, as the negative bone-to-tooth discrepancy that caused them to be retained in this position was a causal factor of high prevalence in both females and males.

In the case of the association of sex with the treatment of tooth retention, there was no dependency relationship either, as both females and males were more likely to use tooth extraction as the most frequently implemented treatment variant, as well as orthodontic treatment. No research was found that addressed this relationship. I believe that this is due to the fact that the therapeutic options are independent of sex, since in order to choose the appropriate therapeutic management, it is essential to take into account factors such as age, tooth position and the systemic state of the patient, for which a careful evaluation of the state of development of the dentition and the assessment of risk agents are essential in order to avoid dental sequelae at a later age. It is important to establish this relationship because it is very common for girls to come to the orthodontic clinic with retained teeth for treatment, due to a greater aesthetic concern, however this research shows that the male sex had a higher prevalence in this regard.

CONCLUSIONS

- The sex most affected by tooth retention was male, with a mean age of 11.4 years, while in females it was 12.1 years.
- Canines were the most commonly retained teeth and in vestibular position.
- Persistent rainstorm and negative bone-tooth discrepancy were the most frequent causes.
- Extraction of the gale was the most widely implemented treatment.
- No sex-dependent relationship with the position and treatment of the impacted tooth was reported in the statistical analysis.

RERENCIASBIBLIOGRÁFICAS

1. Rodríguez Licea ED, Rodríguez Rosales NL, Labrada Ramírez NE. Multidisciplinary treatment of a retained tooth. Presentation of a case. Revméd Granma. Multimed [Internet]April 2019 [cited 26 May 2023]; 23(2):47-354.Available from: http://scielo.sld.cu/scielo.php?script=sci arttext&pid=S1028-48182019000200347&lng=en

2. Fundora Moreno DA, Rodríguez Corbo AA, Corbo Rodríguez MT, et al. Characterization of patients operated on for dental retention in Pinar del Río, 2017-2018. Revista Científica Estudiantil de Cienfuegos Inmedsur [Internet] 2020 [cited: 26 May 2023]; 3(1):9-14.Available from: http://www.inmedsur.cfg.sld.cu/index.php/inmedsur/article/view/55.

3. Pentón García V, Véliz Águila Z, Herrera L. Retained-inverted tooth. Case report: diagnostic and evaluation models. Medisur [Internet]2009Dic.[citado04Abr2024];7(6):59-63.Disponibleen:

   http:// scielo.sld. cu/scielo.php?script=sci arttext&pid=S1727-897X2009000600010&lng=en.

4. Robalino León GV, Martínez Hernández EA, Herrera Navarrete IS, et al. Orthodontic management of retained upper central incisors in patients with cleft palate. Rev Mex Ortodon[Internet] 2020 [cited 29January 2024];8(1):16-22.Available from:https://www.medigraphic.com/cgi-bin/new/resumen.cgi?IDARTICULO =102848

5. González Espangler L. Anatomoradiographic characteristics of third molars in pre-university adolescents. Rev Cub Estomatología [Internet] 2019[cited 29 January 2024]; 56(2)e1722:1-14.Available from:https://www.medigraphic.com/pdfs/revcubest/esc-2019/esc192e.pdf

6. Diaz E. Horizontally retained central incisor. Clinical management. Revista Electrónica de Portales Medicos.com[Internet]18February,2018. [Cited on

   13/06/2023]. Available at: https://www.revista-portalesmedicos.com/revista-medica/incisivo-central-retenidohorizontalmente-manejo-clinico/

7. Márquez Lizárraga AP, Soto Castro TA. Orthodontic treatment in patients with retained canines. RevistaTamé[Internet]2020.8(22),895- 898. Cited February 09, 2024, from https://www.medigraphic.com/pdfs/tame/tam2019/tam1922l.pdf.

8. Rodríguez Díaz AM, Pérez Alfonso A, Toledo Pimentel B. Dental retention of the right upper central incisor due to compound odontoma". I Jornada Virtual de Estomatología 2022. Ciego de Avila [Internet] 2021. [Cited on 13/06/2023].Available at: https://estocavila2021.sld.cu/index.php/estocavila/2022/paper/view/28/52

9. Jiménez RY, Coca GRM, Durán MD. Supernumerary teeth and multiple retention. Review of the literature and presentation of a patient. Acta Med Cent. 2017;

11(2):58-63. [Cited 13/06/2023].Available at: https://www.medigraphic.com/cgi-in/new/resumen.cgi?IDARTICULO=71454.

10. Flores Flores DA, López Cavazos E, Vértix Félix K, etal. Orthodontic-surgical management of a retained lower permanent central incisor. Odontol Pediátr;29(3):146-156 [Internet] 2021.[Cited on 13/06/2023].Available at: https://www.odontologiapediatrica.com/wp-content/uploads/2022/01/5 NC385-OdontologiaPediatrica-V29N3-V4-WEB.pdf

11. Cruz Celi RJ. Frequency of ectopic eruption of upper and lower permanent first molars in children aged 6 to 9 years seen at the clinic of the Universidad César Vallejo from June to September 2019 in the city of Piura-Perí. [Doctoral thesis] Chiclayo: Universidad Católica Santo Toribio de Mogrovejo [Internet] 2019; p.15. [cited 16 December 2023] Available from: http://tesis.usat.edu.pe/handle/20.500.12423/2643.

12. Castillo Alcoser CM, Crespo Mora VI. Most frequent stages of eruption and position of third molars included. Riobamba 2019. Research work for the degree of Odontologist. 2019; p9 [Internet] Jun 2019 [cited 4 Apr 2024].Available from: http://dspace.unach.edu.ec/handle/51000/5766.

13. Moncayo JP. Management of late dental eruption. Degree work prior to obtaining the degree of Odontologist. University of Guayaquil. October 2020; p13 [cited 4 Apr 2024] Available from: http://repositorio.ug.edu.ec/bitstream/redug/49750/1/3480MONCAYOjean.pdff

14. Alvarado Rodríguez N. Prevalence of dental retention in primary and permanent dentition. University of Guayaquil. Pilot Faculty of Dentistry. Ecuador [internet] April 2022 [cited 2023 Jan 29]:1-75. Available from: http://repositorio.ug.edu.ec/bitstream/redug/60591/1/3977/ALVARADOnathaly.pdf

15. De la Cruz Sedano G, Ventura Flores A, Jara Porroa J, et al. Dental eruption:

molecular basis. A review article. Rev Cient Odontol (Lima) 2020; 8(1): e009. [cited 2023 Jan 29] Available from: https://revistas.cientifíca.edu.pe/index.php/odontologica/article/view/606.

16. Hernández CL, Pérez PDT, Fernández QY, et al. Chronology and sequence of permanent dental eruption in children aged 5 to 12 years. Salud ciencia tec. [Internet] 2021; 1(1). [cited 2023 Jan 29] Available from: https://www.medigraphic.com/cgibin/new/resumen.cgi?IDARTICULO=106966.

17. Gil de la Serna L, Melero Alarcón C, Martínez Basse S, et al. Update of the second 21 molar-included seconds etiological factors.Revista Puesta al día [Internet] November 2019; 14 (2): p.123- 128. [cited 18 December 2023] Available from: https://coem.org.es/pdf/publicaciones/cientifica/vol14num2/factoresEtiologicos.pdf

18. Escoda CG, Aytes LB. Tratado de Cirugía buccal tomo I. Inclusion of teeth. Therapeutic possibilities in the case of dental occlusion. 2011. Madrid: Ergon; p.341 [Internet] [Cited 20 January 2023]. Available at: https://gravepa.com/granaino/biblioteca/publicacionesmedicas/Odontologia %20and%20Estomatologia/cirugía/Tratado De Cirugía Buccal - Tomo I.pdf.

19. Hernández D. Oral surgery. Retained teeth[Internet]2021[Cited on 13/06/2023].Available at: http://uvsfajardo.sld.cu/sites/uvsfajardo.sld.cu/files/dientes retenidos.pdf

20. Segura Domínguez GM. Prevalence of retained anterior teeth in paediatric patients. University of Guayaquil. Pilot Faculty of Dentistry. Ecuador [Internet]18June2020 [cited 26 May 2023]:1-76. Available from:

http://repositorio.ug.edu.ec/bitstream/redug/48323/1/SEGURAgabriela3340.pdf

21. Álvarez Mora I, Rivas Pérez G, Morera Pérez A, et al. Orthodontic-surgical treatment in a patient with a retained canine. Case presentation. X Simposio Visión Salud Bucal y IX Taller sobre el Cáncer Bual2021.Universidad de Ciencias Médicas de Cienfuegos [Internet] 2021[cited 26 May 2023]:1-76.Available in:

http ://estomatovision2021. sld. cu/index.php/estomatovision/2021/paper/view/165.

22. Díaz Palomino SY. Retained canine in the upper jaw. Work of professional sufficiency for the professional title of dental surgeon. Perú 2020 [cited 8 May 023] Available from: https://repositorio.upla.edu.pe/handle /20.500.12848/1827

23. Rivero Pérez O. Oral surgery. Selection of topics. Editorial Ciencias Médicas.

Havana 2018, p.233-256.

24. Quevedo Aliaga JL, Mas Torres M, Mayedo Nuñez Y, et al. Local causes of retained permanent canines in patients of the René Guzmán Pérez Stomatological Clinic of Calixto García. CCH Correo cient Holguín [Internet] Jul-Sep 2017 [cited 26 May 2023]; 21(3): 627-636. Available from: http://scielo.sld.cu/scielo.php?pid=S1560- 43812017000300002&script=sci arttext&tlng=pt

25. Perero López KS. Local factors causing retention of canine teeth in the maxilla: A literature review. [Degree thesis]. Guayaquil: University of Guayaquil. [Internet] 2019; p.26-43 [cited 2023 Feb 15]. Available from: http://repositorio.ug.edu.ec/bitstream/redug/33808/1/2691PEREROkatherine .pdf

26. Echegaray Soria GC. Aetiological factors causing retention of permanent canines. [Degree thesis]. Guayaquil: University of Guayaquil. [Internet] 2021; p.23-27 [cited 10 February 2023]. Available from:

http ://repositorio.ug. edu. ec/bitstream/redug/51666/1/3614ECHEGARAY gary .pdf

27. Guirola Rodríguez I. Included canines. Update on their management in primary health care. Research project prior to obtaining a degree in dentistry. San Gregorio de Portoviejo University. [Internet] 2020; p13 [cited 10 February 2023]. Available from: http://repositorio.sangregorio.edu.ec. /handle/123456789/2703.

28. Cushpa Pilco CX. Diagnostic characterisation of the dental treatment of adolescents with retained canines. Degree dissertation for the title of Dentist. Riobamba. Ecuador [Internet] 2023; p 23 [cited 10 February 2023]. Available from: http://dspace.unach.edu.ec/handle/51000/12015.

29. Yllarreta Bandera M, Guerra Cobián O, Leiva Lima L. Concurrent occurrence of complex odontoma and dentigerous cyst associated with tooth retention. Medicentro Electrónica [Internet]2020 Dec.[cited2024Apr 05]; 24(4): 833-841. Available from: http://scielo.sld.cu/scielo.php?script=sci arttext&pid=S1029-30432020000400833&lng=en.

30. Blanco Ruiz Y, Biblioni Serra L, Espinosa Morales L. Prevention of permanent canine retention in the paediatric and juvenile population. Odontosantiago [Internet] 2023 [cited 5 Apr 2024]. Available from:

http:// odontosantiago. sld. cu/index.php/odontosantiago/2023/paper/download

/19/48.

31. Félix Morales GC. Prevalence of included permanent teeth and their degree of inclination with respect to the occlusal plane of patients integrated into the Dr. René Puig Bentz Dentistry Clinic, period January 2018-2019. Degree thesis for the degree of Dentist [Internet] 2019 [cited 5 Apr 2024] Available from: http://repositorio.unphu.edu.do/handle/123456789/3464.

32. Sánchez Velásquez J, Molina Barahona M. Retained canines, clinical characteristics, diagnostic methods and dental treatment. Bibliographic review. Odontol. Act. [Internet]. Sep 5, 2022 [cited 5 Apr 2024];7(3): 65-74. Available from: http://oactiva.ucacue.edu.ec/index.php/oactiva/article/view/700.

33. Mercado Portal J, Mamani Cahuata L. Assessment of the space available for the eruption of the lower third molar included according to the mandibular side using panoramic radiographs in patients aged 17 to 36 years at the Ceden Puno 2021 clinic. Thesis project [Internet] [cited 5 Apr 2024]. Available from: http://vriunap.pe/fedu/upload/2021/p00000527-4-Proy.pdf.

34. Gorriz MC de S, Cianca LOA, Bertram CEA, et al. Cleidocranial dysplasia - a family case report. J Multidiscip Dent [Internet] March 4, 2024 [cited April 5, 2024]; 11(3):162-6. Available from: https://jmdentistry.com/jmd/article/view/896

35. Aquino Lozada CA. Diagnosis in Orthodontics. Integration of a clinical case. Thesis for the degree of Dental Surgeon. Universidad Nacional Autónoma de México [Internet] August 2021. p80 [cited 5 Apr 2024]. Disponible en: https://ru.dgb.unam.mx/bitstream/20.500.14330/TES01000813948/3/0813948.pdf

36. Hernández García A. Surgical-orthodontic approach to dental inclusions with orthodontic buttons. Thesis for the degree of Dental Surgeon. Nacional Autónoma de México [Internet]September2023.p12.[cited 5 Apr 2024]. Disponible en: https://ru.dgb.unam.mx/bitstream/20.500.14330/TES01000846643/3/0846643.pdf

37. Grybiene V, Juozénaité D, Kubiliuté K. Diagnostic methods and treatment strategies of impacted maxillary canines: a review of the literature. PubMed [Internet]2019; 21(1): p. 3-12. [cited 22 Feb.

2023]Available at: https://pubmed.ncbi.nlm.nih.gov/31619657/

38. Gallardo CP, Contreras CC, Quezada AS, et al. Contribution of oral and maxillofacial radiology to clinical diagnosis. Advances in Odontostomatology, March 2019. 35(2); 73-82. [Internet].[cited 22 Feb. 2023] Available from:

http://scielo.isciii.es/pdf/odonto/v35n2/0213-1285-odonto-35-2-73.pdf.

39. Ramírez LB, Chacón VR, Rivas AH. The use of X-rays in dentistry and the importance of the justification of radiographic examinations. Advances in Odontostomatology [Internet] 2020; 36(3); 131-142. [cited 2023 Feb 22] Available from:http://scielo.isciii.es/pdf/odonto/v36n3/0213-1285-odonto-36-3- 131.pdf.

40. Carballido Ferreira E. Diagnosis of canine included. World's Hygienist. Madrid professional association of dental hygienists[Internet]August 14, 2019. [cited 10 March 2023]. Available from: http://colegiohigienistasmadrid.org/blog/?p=213.

41. Cabanillas MD, Vásquez BD. Análisis de la variabilidad de la configuración interna de condutos radiculares de los premolares mediante tomografía computarizadaCONE-BEAM.UniversidadPrivadaAntonioGuillermoUrrelo, Facultad de Ciencias de la Salud. Cajamarca Perú [Internet] 2020 [cited March 10, 2023].Available from: http://repositorio.upagu.edu.pe/handle/UPAGU/1453

42. Ruiz Imbert AC, Cascante Sequeira D. Grayscale density values in Cone Beam Computed Tomography: scope and limitations [Internet] 2021. ODOVTOS-Int.J.DentalSc.23(2);167-176. [cited 10 March 2023]. Available from: http://www.medigraphic.com/cgi- bin/new/summary.cgi?IDARTICLE=104260.

43. Ticona Apaza V. Cone Beam tomography in the identification of third molars with proximity to the lower dental canal. Speciality Thesis. Universidad Mayor de San Andrés. La Paz, Bolivia.[Internet]2023[cited 10 March 2024].

Available at: http://repositorio.umsa.bo/handle/123456789/35058.

44. Márquez Conde A. Prevalence of retained teeth in a sample of the population of San Luis Potosí analysed by CBCT tomography. Master's thesis. Universidad Autónoma de San Luis Potosí [Internet] July 2021 [cited 10 March 2024]. Available from: http://repositorioinstitucional.uaslp.mx/xmlui/handle/i/7871

45. Trujillo Fandiño JJ. Tooth retention in the anterior region. Dental practice 1990:29-35.

46. Ugalde Morales FJ, González LR. Prevalence of canine impaction in patients treated at the UNITEC orthodontic clinic. Rev ADM; 56(2):49-58. [Internet] 1999 [cited 10 March 2024]. Available from: https://www.medigraphic.com/cgi-bin/new/resumen.cgi?IDARTICULO=9608

47. Blanco Ruiz Y, Bibiloni Serra L, Espinosa Morales L. Prevention of permanent

canine retention in the infant and juvenile population. I International Congress. Cuban Society of Stomatological Sciences. Santiago de Cuba Chapter.[Internet]June2023[cited20January2024]. Available from http://odontosantiago.sld.cu/index.php/odontosantiago/2023/paper/download/19/48 .

48. Pichel Borges I, Suárez García MC, González Espangler L, et al. Dental retention in orthodontic patients aged 8 to 18 years. Rev16 April. [Internet] 17 March 2018[cited 26 May 2023]; 57(268):89-96.Available from: http://www.rev16deabril.sld.cu/index.php/16-04/article/download/613/279

49. Restrepo JD, Mariaca PB. Management and periodontal prognosis of retained canines in orthodontics. Universidad Cooperativa de Colombia [Internet] 2019;1-22.[cited26May2023].Available from: https://repository.ucc.edu.co/bitstream/20.500.12494/13947/6/2019 pronostico periodontal retenidos.pdf

50. Miranda Silva A, Villacís Pérez D, López Seda D, et al. Included canines, dental treatment: literature review. Revista Latinoamericana de Ortodoncia y Odontopediatría [Internet].5December2020;35(2) [cited 2023 December 17]. Available from: https://www.ortodoncia.ws/publicaciones/2020/art-53/

51. Proaño Silva JC. Imaging diagnosis and clinical treatment of retained canine. Degree thesis. University of Guayaquil. Pilot Faculty of Dentistry [Internet] August 2019; p 23 [cited 5 March 2023]. Available from: http://repositorio.ug.edu.ec/handle/redug/44283

52. Macías Escalada E, Cobo Plana J, Carlos Villafranca F, et al. Surgical orthodontic approach to dental inclusions. RCOE [Internet]Feb 2005 [cited 9 Jul 2023];10(1):69-82. Available from: http://scielo.isciii.es/scielo.php?script=sci arttext&pid=S1138-123X2005000100006

53. Díaz Guerra Y, Cuyac Lantigua M. Importance of prevention in stomatology from school age. Rev Méd Electrón. [Internet] Jul 2022 [44(4):754-757cited 6 Jun 2023]; Available from: http://scielo.sld.cu/scielo.php?pid=S1684182420220004007548&script=sci arttext&tln g=pt.

54. Lovo J. Quaternary prevention: towards a new paradigm. Aten Fam. [Internet] 2020 27 (4):212-215. [cited 6 Jun 2023]; Available from: https://www.medigraphic.com/cgibin/new/resumen.cgi?IDARTICULO=95859

55. Ovalle Y, Pac G, Barrios R. Medicina preventiva y niveles de prevención Guatemala: Universidad de San Carlos de Guatemala[Internet]2019 [cited 6 Jun 2023].Available from: http://www.medicina.cunoc.edu.gt/articulos/ab79b79d062738543b4086f16b9454f93d cfc81f.pdf

56. Cárdenas Suárez LE, Carpio Vaca GA, Humala Rojas JX, et al. Health promotion and prevention in society. Tesla Revista Científica [Internet] 2021 [cited 6 Jun 2023]. Available from:

http s ://tesla.puertomaderoeditorial.com.ar/index.php/tesla/article/ view/21

57. Couto Assis W, Santos Pereira J, Santos-Silva Y, et al. Factors associated with malocclusion in preschool children in a small Brazilian city.PesquiBrasOdontopediatriaClínIntegr[Internet]202020:e5351 .[cited 6 Jun 2023];Available from:

https://www.scielo.br/j/pboci/a/qYY4NBKmRh3fMHSkRMxNqSG/?format=html &la ng=en

58. Ganapathi A, Jeevanandan J. Parental Awareness About Malocclusion in Their Children in Chennai Population .International Journal of Pharmaceutical Research [Internet] 2020 [cited 6 Jun 2023]; 12(3):2669- 2681.Available from: https://www.researchgate.net/profile/GaneshJeevanandan2/publication/344757952 Pa rental Pa rental Awareness About Malocclusion in Their Children in Chennai Population/l inks/5f9d837d299bf1b53e548b32/Parental-Awareness-AboutMalocclusion-in-Their- Children-in-Chennai-Population.pdf.

59. Nerurkar S, Kamble R. Comparative assessment of the need for preventive and interceptive orthodontic treatment in 6,9 and 12 year old children in central India. F1000Research [Internet] 2023[cited 6 Jun 2023]; 12:472. Available from: https://f1000research.com/articles/12-472

60. Román Chaguay YF. Prevalence of retained canines in the Mc Sthetic Dental Office. Guayaquil: Universidad de Guayaquil [Internet] 2020 [cited 6 Jun 2023]. Available from: http://repositorio.ug.edu.ec/handle/redug/48507

61. Mendoza Rodríguez M, Rodríguez Sierra O, Medina Solís CE, et al. Prevalence of retained canines in patients attending ICSa. Educ Salud Bol Científico Inst Cienc Salud Univ Autónoma Estado Hidalgo.8(16);14-19. [Internet] 2020 [cited 16 October 2023]. Available from: https://repository.uaeh.edu.mx/revistas/index.php/ICSA/issue/archive).

62. González Espangler L, Ramírez Quevedo Y, Durán Vázquez WE, et al. Presence of third molars in the Policlínico José Martí. Proceedings of the International Congress of Stomatology; 2015 Nov; Havana City. Cuba [Internet] 2015[cited 26 Mar 23]. Available from:

http://www.estomatologia2015.sld.cu/index.php/estomatologia/nov2015/paper/view/6 45/406

63. Pérez J. Causes and incidences of retention in permanent canines: Literature review. [Undergraduate Thesis]Ecuador: Universidad de Guayaquil [Internet] 2018 [cited 26 Mar 23] Available from: http://repositorio.ug.edu.ec/handle/redug/29552.

64. Suárez Gargate J. Prevalence of retained teeth in patients aged 15 to 60 years seen at the Cero Huánuco radiology centre [Internet] 2018 [cited 26 Mar 23].Available from:

https://alicia.concytec.gob.pe/vufind/Record/UDHR 2ee4ad16698020fcd9d284270 65abf7c/

65. Ayala Pérez Y, Carralero Zaldívar L, Leyva Ayala B. Dental eruption and its influencing factors. Correo Científico Médico [Internet] 2018 [cited 7 Apr 2024];

22 (4) Available at: https://revcocmed.sld.cu/index.php/cocmed/article/view/2931

66. Quisbert Laura JZ. Aetiology and incidence in the retention of permanent canines. Degree work for the title of Specialist in Orthodontics and Dento Maxillofacial Orthopaedics. Bolivia [Internet] 2022 [cited 16 October 2023] Available from: http://repositorio.umsa.bo/xmlui/handle/123456789/29828

67. Leal Becerra CL, Rodríguez Cotrina NM. Frequency of retained canines in patients aged 14 to 20 years, period 2017 - 2019, Cajamarca. Thesis for the Professional Title of Dental Surgeon. Peru [internet] 2021 [Cited 27 July 2023]. Available from: http://repositorio.upagu.edu.pe/handle/UPAGU/1830.

68. Quintana Díaz JC, Algozain Acosta Y, Quintana Giralt M et al. Surgical treatment of retained teeth in the maxillofacial surgery service of Artemisa (1994-2010).RevActaOdontolCol2015[cited20Sep2023]; 5(1):57-63.Availableat:https://repositorio.unal.edu.co/handle/unal/61368

69. Diaz P, Sue Y. Retained maxillary canine. Peruvian University Los

Andes [internet2020] [cited 20 Sep 2023] Available from: https://repositorio.upla.edu.pe/handle/20.500.12848/1827.

70. Corrales A. Orthodontic-surgical treatment of retained canines in a 14-year-old patient. Pinar del Rio Medical Journal, 965-972. [Internet] 2019 [cited Jan 10, 2023]. Retrieved fromhttp://scielo.sld.cu/pdf7rpr/v22n5/rpr15518.pdf

71. Cornejo Meléndez M. Prevalence of retained lower canines in panoramic radiographs of patients aged 15 to 24 years at the UCSM dental centre, period 2022-2023. Catholic University of San Martin. Peru [Internet] 2023. Available at: https://repositorio.ucsm.edu.pe/handle/20.500.12920/13149.

ANNEXES

Participant observation

Annex 3:

Objectives:

- o Obtain information on the variables and radiographic aspects of interest for the research.

Aspects to observe in the patient

- ■ General patient data, especially sex, age, personal and family history, habits.
- ■ Extra oral examination: maxillary sinusitis, alopecia, exophthalmos.
- ■ Intraoral examination: absence of the tooth past the age of eruption, persistence of primary teeth, clinical manifestations of cysts or tumours, alterations in the lateral incisors, supernumerary teeth and/or crowding, anomalies of shape and size of the teeth, central diastema, submucosal fibrosis, changes in the colour of the mucosa covering the retained tooth (ischaemia, erythema), haematomas, pain, hypoaesthesia, trauma.

Aspects to be observed in the X-rays:

- o Bone density.
- o Depth of impaction in relation to the occlusal plane.
- o Direction of eruption and angle of inclination of the tooth.
- o Length, shape and direction of roots.
- o Shape and size of the crown
- o Periodontal ligament space
- o Ankylosis
- o Hypercementosis
- o Radiolucent lesions in relation to the retained tooth (chistenedentigerous, root cyst of a deciduous tooth, odontoma)

Annex 4

Form

Objective: To collect the variables of interest for this research.

Aspects to be taken into account:

1. Sex:

Female Male

2. Age:
3. **Location of the retained incisor:**

Unilateral

Upper right

Upper left Bilateral

Lower right Top

Lower left

Location of the impacted canine Inferior

Unilateral Bilateral

Upper right Upper

Upper left Lower

Lower right

Lower left

4. Position of the retained tooth

VestibularLingual PalatineMiddle

5. Causes of retention: (Local)

Irregular tooth position or pressure from an adjacent tooth

Supernumerary teeth

Persistence of the storm

Gingival fibrosis

Bone density

Chronic non-infectious inflammation

Bone-tooth discrepancy negative

Cystic and tumour disease: root cyst of a deciduous tooth, dentigerous cyst, odontoma

Infectious disease

Alveolar tooth trauma

Systemic:

Prenatal causes:

Hereditary and genetic

_________ Congenital

Mixed breeds

Postnatal:

_________ AnaemiaMalnutritionSyphilis

_________ ScurvyTuberculosisBeri Beri

Endocrine dysfunctionHypothyroidism ,

Early sexual development

Rare conditions:

Cleidocranial dysplasia,

Crouzon Syndrome

6. Treatment of choice

_________ Abstention

_________ Extraction

Orthodontic treatment

Orthodontic-surgical treatment

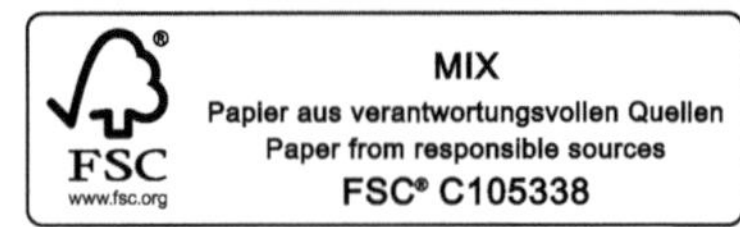

Printed by Books on Demand GmbH, Norderstedt / Germany